Type 2 Diabetes

All you need to know

Dr. Sheila Harrison

Disclaimer

This content is not a substitute for consulting a professional physician but to give a fair knowledge about the disease and to equip you to seek medical assistance as early as possible if need be to avoid complications. It should also be noted that the area of medical science is a constantly changing field and due to the ever developing and changing nature of medical knowledge, we suggest you seek expert advice if you spot any discrepancies or decide to take action in reaction to the information in this content. Never reject medical advice from professionals or put off getting treatment because of something you read online, acquired through this material, or any other online resource.

And remember the internet won't heal you but God through Physicians will.

Table of Content

Introduction

A major public health problem with significant effects on both individuals and society, type 2 diabetes is on the rise globally. When the body's capacity to regulate blood sugar levels is weakened, it manifests as a severe metabolic disease. Elevated glucose levels are the effect of this.

Over the last few decades, the prevalence of type 2 diabetes has increased as a result of factors like sedentary lifestyles, poor dietary decisions, and genetic susceptibility. Its effects go beyond physical health, as it also plays a role in a number of consequences like cardiovascular disease, renal problems, and neuropathy. Understanding the underlying processes and practical treatment techniques is crucial given its prevalence and related difficulties.

Chronic hyperglycemia, or an excessive quantity of glucose circulating in the blood plasma, is a feature of type 2 diabetes. This happens as a result of high blood sugar levels brought on by insulin resistance and incorrect insulin production. Complex interplay between genetic, environmental, and lifestyle variables play a role in the etiology of this disease.

Section 1

What distinguishes type 1 from type 2 diabetes?

Elevated blood sugar levels are a typical characteristic of both type 1 and type 2 diabetes. But they have different underlying causes. The immune system of the body assaults and kills insulin-producing beta cells in the pancreas in type 1 diabetes, an autoimmune disease. Due to the complete lack of insulin, lifelong insulin replacement treatment is necessary. Type 2 diabetes, on the other hand, often manifests later in life and is defined by insulin resistance, in which the body's cells stop responding to insulin. In addition, reduced insulin secretion is frequently observed over time. Both forms of diabetes need to be managed carefully, but because they have different underlying causes and processes, they call for different strategies.

Section 2

What percentage of people have type 2 diabetes?

The prevalence of type 2 diabetes has reached epidemic levels around the world, making it one of the most important issues in contemporary public health. Because of alterations in lifestyle, urbanization, and aging populations, it is more common now. Over 37 million Americans (roughly 1 in 10) have diabetes, and 90–95% of them have type 2, according to the CDC. The majority of persons with type 2 diabetes are over the age of 45, but it is becoming more common among kids, teenagers, and young adults. If current trends continue, it is expected that by 2045, there will be over 90 million individuals worldwide who have diabetes.

Significant geographical differences can be seen in the prevalence of type 2 diabetes. Since rapid urbanization and nutritional changes have increased the burden of obesity and sedentary lifestyles, it is more common in low- and middle-income nations. On the other hand, because unhealthy lifestyles are so common, the frequency is still high in high-income nations.

Section 3

What effects does the rise in type 2 diabetes cases have?

Numerous socioeconomic and health system issues brought on by the rising incidence of type 2 diabetes present difficulties for both individuals and society as a whole.

- **Healthcare costs:** The economic burden of type 2 diabetes is substantial, driven by the costs of medical care, medications, and management of diabetes-related complications. This burden is shouldered not only by individuals but also by healthcare systems and governments. The costs extend beyond direct medical expenses to include indirect costs, such as lost productivity and disability.

- **Impact on quality of life:** Individuals living with type 2 diabetes face a reduced quality of life due to the physical, psychological, and social challenges posed by the condition and its complications. The need for continuous self-management, dietary restrictions, and the risk of complications like cardiovascular disease, neuropathy, and retinopathy contribute to a diminished quality of life.

- **Health disparities:** Socioeconomic factors play a significant role in the prevalence and management of type 2 diabetes. Vulnerable populations, including those with limited access to healthcare, lower socioeconomic status, and educational disparities, are at a higher risk of developing the condition and experiencing worse outcomes. Addressing health disparities is crucial for equitable diabetes prevention and management.

- **Healthcare systems strain:** The increasing prevalence of type 2 diabetes places immense pressure on healthcare systems worldwide. The demand for diabetes-related care, including regular monitoring, medication, and specialized interventions, strains healthcare resources and facilities. Integrated and multidisciplinary approaches are required to effectively manage the growing burden.

Section 4

What are the causes of type 2 diabetes?

Type 2 diabetes is brought on by a number of variables. They include risk factors linked to ethnicity, family history, genetic predisposition, and aging. Type 2 diabetes is largely caused by genetic factors, which also affect susceptibility to the disease. According to evidence, diabetes has a genetic component and is more likely to affect those who have a family history of the disease. Specific genetic variations that alter insulin production, insulin sensitivity, and other metabolic pathways have been found to affect type 2 diabetes risk.

Numerous of these genetic variations are linked to insulin resistance and beta-cell malfunction, two factors that are crucial for the onset of type 2 diabetes. It's crucial to realize that a person does not necessarily need to be genetically predisposed to develop diabetes. Environmental variables, such as lifestyle decisions, have a large role as well.

Family history and ethnicity's roles A recognized risk factor for the disease is having a family history of type 2 diabetes. One's chance of getting diabetes increases if they have a first-degree relative (parent, sibling, or other close family) who has the disease. This shows a complicated interaction between a family's shared environmental influences and genetic predisposition.

Additionally, ethnicity affects diabetes risk. A greater susceptibility to type 2 diabetes exists among several ethnic groups, including African Americans, Hispanic Americans, Native Americans, and South Asians. This might be a result of a variety of genetic, cultural, nutritional, and socioeconomic health variables that differ among various ethnic communities.

Section 5

What is the medical science behind Type 2 diabetes?

Intricate pathophysiological processes underpinning type 2 diabetes include oxidative damage, chronic inflammation, insulin resistance, and beta-cell malfunction.

Insulin refractoriness Type 2 diabetes is characterized by insulin resistance, which is defined by a reduced ability of target tissues (such as muscle, liver, and adipose tissue) to respond to the effects of insulin. The body's capacity to control the intake and use of glucose is interfered with by this resistance, which raises blood sugar levels. Insulin resistance is exacerbated by the adipokines and cytokines secreted by adipose tissue, particularly visceral fat. In order to make up for this problem, the pancreas must create more insulin, which eventually exhausts the beta cells and impairs their ability to regulate glucose.

The cause of type 2 diabetes is heavily influenced by beta-cell dysfunction and decreased insulin production. Over time, beta-cell malfunction and decreased insulin output might result from elevated insulin demand brought on by insulin resistance. Additionally, beta-cell survival and function can be hampered by long-term exposure to high blood glucose levels. As a result, the pancreas is less able to react to variations in blood sugar levels appropriately, which exacerbates hyperglycemia.

Diabetes-related chronic low-grade inflammation: Inflammation is the body's method of responding to issues, such as when you receive a cut and your skin swells and gets red. But occasionally, such as in type 2 diabetes, there is an inflammation that is difficult to treat. This chronic inflammation plays a significant role in why diabetes worsens. It takes place as a result of the body's fat releasing problematic substances. These substances hinder the correct functioning of the hormone insulin, which causes issues with blood sugar levels. Additionally, this inflammation causes the body to produce substances that hinder insulin's effectiveness. Additionally, this inflammation disrupts how certain cells function in a particular area of the body.

Cellular damage and oxidative stress: Oxidative stress is similar to a health issue for the body. Reactive oxygen species, which are like small troublemakers, and antioxidants, which are like helpers that mend things, are out of balance, which causes it to occur. Type 2 diabetes can result in cell damage from this issue.

This issue arises when there is an abundance of sugar and fatty substances in the body. The pancreas, blood arteries, and nerves are just a few of the bodily organs that might be harmed by this issue. Additionally, it hinders the effectiveness of insulin and increases inflammation, which exacerbates diabetes.

Section 6

What are the risk factors of type 2 diabetes?

Environmental effects, lifestyle decisions, obesity-related issues, and demographic traits are all included in the risk factors.

Age as a risk factor for type 2 diabetes: Age is a significant risk factor. Although the illness can appear at any age, being older increases the chance. This is partially a result of the deteriorating insulin sensitivity that frequently comes with aging, changes in body composition, and decreased physical activity. The pancreas' capacity to produce insulin may also decline with age, which might exacerbate the progression of diabetes.

Due to its frequency among older people, type 2 diabetes was once known as adult-onset diabetes. But with the growth in sedentary behavior and juvenile obesity, type 2 diabetes diagnoses in kids and teens have alarmingly increased, necessitating a change in nomenclature.

Environment-related factors Environmental elements are very important in the emergence of type 2 diabetes. Modern lifestyles marked by simple availability to high-calorie, low-nutrient meals and sedentary habits considerably contribute to the condition's increased prevalence. An atmosphere that encourages unhealthy eating habits, such as excessive intake of processed foods and sugary drinks, raises the risk of obesity and insulin resistance, both of which are essential components in the emergence of type 2 diabetes.

Metabolic syndrome and obesity: Type 2 diabetes is greatly increased by being overweight. Adipose tissue that is too abundant, particularly visceral or abdominal fat, causes cells to become less susceptible to the effects of insulin. In order to manage blood sugar levels, the pancreas must create more insulin, which eventually exhausts the beta cells and impairs glucose regulation. The risk of type 2 diabetes is further increased by metabolic syndrome, a collection of disorders that includes obesity, high blood pressure, abnormal lipid profiles, and raised blood sugar.

Sedentary behavior and lack of physical exercise: Sedentary behavior and a lack of physical activity are major risk factors for type 2 diabetes. Regular exercise supports weight loss, improves metabolic health overall, and helps to increase insulin sensitivity. On the other hand, a sedentary lifestyle encourages weight gain, messes with glucose control, and raises the possibility of metabolic dysfunction.

Demographic variables such as gender, ethnic predilection, and gestational diabetes can also affect the likelihood of acquiring type 2 diabetes. Men are often at higher risk than women, and this is influenced by gender. The danger does, however, increase as people become older. Additionally, because of a mix of genetic vulnerability and cultural/environmental variables, several ethnic groups, including African Americans, Hispanic Americans, Native Americans, and some Asian communities, have a higher tendency to type 2 diabetes.

Another risk factor is gestational diabetes, a kind of diabetes that appears during pregnancy.

Type 2 diabetes is more likely to strike women who have gestational diabetes in the future. Their children are also at risk, demonstrating the intergenerational effects of diabetes risk.

Section 7

What are the symptoms of type 2 diabetes?

Type 2 diabetes can manifest itself in many different ways clinically. There are a few typical symptoms, nevertheless, that people could encounter. These include increased appetite (polyphagia), frequent urination (polyuria), unexplained weight loss, and polydipsia, which is excessive thirst. However, some people with type 2 diabetes may go for a long time without showing any symptoms, which delays diagnosis.

HbA1c readings, oral glucose tolerance tests, and fasting plasma glucose measurements are used to diagnose type 2 diabetes. Diabetes is defined by the American Diabetes Association (ADA) as having a fasting plasma glucose level below 126 mg/dL (7.0 mmol/L), a two-hour plasma glucose level below 200 mg/dL (11.1 mmol/L), or a HbA1c level below 6.5%. These standards aid in identifying those who need assistance in controlling their blood sugar levels.

Cardiovascular Illness An increased risk of cardiovascular disease is linked to type 2 diabetes. Diabetes increases a person's risk of atherosclerosis, which can cause peripheral arterial disease, coronary artery disease, heart attacks, and strokes. Inflammation, dyslipidemia, chronic hyperglycemia, and insulin resistance all have a role in the onset and progression of various cardiovascular conditions.

The effects of type 2 diabetes on tiny blood arteries and other organs include retinopathy, nephropathy, and neuropathy. The blood vessels in the retina are harmed in diabetic retinopathy, one of the main causes of blindness. Diabetic nephropathy causes inflammation and abnormal blood flow in the kidneys, which may result in kidney failure. Diabetes-related nerve damage known as diabetic neuropathy can cause sensory and motor impairments that affect the limbs and other organs. These issues highlight the need of glycemic management because they are all impacted by persistently high blood sugar levels.

Ulcers on the Diabetic Foot: Neuropathy, peripheral artery dysfunction, and poor wound healing all contribute to diabetic foot problems. Because neuropathy impairs foot feeling, it might be challenging to identify wounds or infections. Blood supply to the feet is restricted by peripheral artery dysfunction, which slows wound healing. These elements working together can result in infections, amputations, and foot ulcers. The key to avoiding these issues is regular foot care and close observation.

Section 8

What are some diagnostic tools and screening for type 2 diabetes?

A persistent issue with how your body uses food for energy is type 2 diabetes. Type 2 diabetes might be challenging occasionally since it does not exhibit obvious symptoms. Finding it early and monitoring it frequently is crucial because of this. Doctors may use a variety of measures to determine if a patient has this form of diabetes or is at risk for developing it thanks to advances in medical understanding.

Fasting Plasma Glucose Test: A typical diagnostic method for determining a person's blood sugar level following an overnight fast is the fasting plasma glucose (FPG) test. In the morning, before any food or liquids are consumed, a blood sample is obtained. Diabetes can be diagnosed if a person's fasting glucose level is 126 mg/dL or above. This examination aids in determining if a person has overt diabetes or pre-diabetes. It gives a snapshot of blood sugar regulation at a given moment in time and is especially helpful for people who might be asymptomatic.

Oral Glucose Tolerance Test: The oral glucose tolerance test (OGTT) is drinking a sweet beverage following an overnight fast, followed by periodic blood sugar level checks. This examination reveals details on how the body metabolizes glucose over time. Diabetes is indicated by a two-hour plasma glucose level of 200 mg/dL or greater during the OGTT. The OGTT is helpful for finding reduced glucose tolerance, another precursor to diabetes, as well as for diagnosing diabetes in cases when fasting glucose readings may not be definitive.

Hemoglobin A1c Measurement: The test of hemoglobin A1c (HbA1c) provides information on the average blood sugar levels over the previous two to three months. The amount of glucose molecules that attach to the hemoglobin in red blood cells is indicated by the HbA1c level. Diabetes is indicated by a HbA1c result of 6.5% or above. Because it doesn't need fasting and gives a longer-term view of blood sugar management, this test is useful. It's especially helpful for people who might struggle with fasting tests or for whom routine testing is prohibitive.

Regular screenings and early diagnosis of type 2 diabetes are important for a number of reasons. First of all, it enables the quick use of management techniques that can greatly postpone or stop the onset of difficulties. Second, early intervention can assist people in making lifestyle changes to better regulate their blood sugar, which can lessen the need for medication and improve general well being.

Equally crucial is routine screening, particularly for those who have risk factors including obesity, a family history of diabetes, or a sedentary lifestyle. Regular screening enables prompt therapies that can stop or slow the evolution of diabetes by identifying pre-diabetes or early stages of the disease.

Section 9

How can type 2 diabetes be managed?

In order to effectively manage type 2 diabetes, a multidimensional strategy is needed that takes into account the condition's many facets, such as blood sugar management, lifestyle changes, and customized treatment programs. We will examine the main type 2 diabetes management techniques in this response.

Diet and exercise: The cornerstone of type 2 diabetes management is lifestyle changes. Dietary modifications are essential for controlling blood sugar levels.

Exercise on a regular basis is equally vital. Exercise boosts cardiovascular health, increases weight loss, and increases insulin sensitivity.

Medications for glycemic control: Medication may be administered if changing one's lifestyle is insufficient to control blood sugar levels. There are several drug classes that focus on various facets of glucose control.

- **Metformin and sulfonylureas:** Metformin is often the first-line medication for type 2 diabetes. It improves insulin sensitivity and reduces glucose production by the liver. Sulfonylureas stimulate insulin secretion from the pancreas. These medications can be effective in lowering blood sugar levels, but they can have side effects such as hypoglycemia and weight gain.

- **Insulin therapy:** Insulin therapy is essential for individuals with advanced type 2 diabetes or when other medications fail to maintain adequate blood sugar control. It helps regulate blood sugar levels by providing the body with the insulin it lacks. Insulin therapy may involve multiple injections or the use of insulin pumps. Regular monitoring and careful dosing adjustments are crucial to preventing hypoglycemia and optimizing glycemic control.

- **GLP-1 receptor agonists:** GLP-1 receptor agonists are injectable medications that mimic the action of GLP-1, a hormone that enhances insulin secretion, slows down digestion, and reduces appetite. These medications can promote weight loss, improve blood sugar control, and have cardiovascular benefits.

- **SGLT-2 inhibitors:** SGLT-2 inhibitors work by blocking the reabsorption of glucose by the kidneys, leading to increased glucose excretion in urine. They also have beneficial effects on blood pressure and weight. These medications are particularly useful for individuals with heart and kidney disease.

Patient-centered approach to treatment selection: Patients and healthcare professionals should work together to determine the best treatment plan. It is important to take into account each person's particular traits, interests, way of life, and medical background. Discussing the advantages, disadvantages, and potential negative effects of various treatment choices with the patient enables them to make educated decisions about their diabetes care. This is known as a patient-centered approach.

Section 10

How can type 2 diabetes be avoided?

While it's possible that your genetics cannot be changed, you can adjust your lifestyle and perhaps lower your chance of having type 2 diabetes. Type 2 diabetes prevention is a crucial public health objective that necessitates a complex strategy that includes both individual and community-based interventions.

Primary prevention strategies: The first step in stopping type 2 diabetes is to address the risk factors that are at the root of the disease. The goal of primary prevention is to stop risk factors from developing in the first place. This entails encouraging active living from an early age, preventing tobacco use, supporting a good diet, and promoting healthy lives overall. People who have prediabetes or are at a high risk of becoming diabetes are the primary focus of primary prevention. A healthy diet and increased physical exercise are two lifestyle changes that are crucial in slowing the development of type 2 diabetes.

Community-wide interventions have a significant influence on avoiding type 2 diabetes, as do health promotion efforts. Collaboration between businesses, workplaces, local governments, and healthcare organizations is crucial. Large-scale behavior change can be influenced by health promotion initiatives that increase knowledge of the value of healthy lifestyles, availability to nutrient-rich foods, and opportunities for physical exercise. The general health of communities can be improved by building surroundings that support healthy choices, such as walking trails and farmers' markets.

High-risk person screening and early intervention: High-risk person screening is a major method for early identification and intervention. It is possible to avoid or delay the onset of diabetes by identifying people with prediabetes or other risk factors in time. In determining risk factors, doing screening tests, and carrying out suitable therapies, healthcare practitioners are essential. In high-risk patients, lifestyle treatments like organized education programs can successfully encourage healthy habits, support weight reduction, and enhance glucose control.

Section 11

FAQ on Type 2 Diabetes

Can type 2 diabetes affect existing kidney diseases?

It may. Type 2 diabetes can lead to diabetic kidney disease, damaging the kidneys' blood vessels and function due to high blood sugar and associated factors like high blood pressure and inflammation. Regular monitoring and managing blood sugar and related factors are essential to prevent or slow this complication.

Can type 2 diabetes affect liver diseases?

It may. Type 2 diabetes can lead to a condition called nonalcoholic fatty liver disease (NAFLD), characterized by excess fat in the liver cells due to insulin resistance and metabolic factors. NAFLD can range from a mild accumulation of fat (NAFL) to inflammation and liver cell damage (NASH), which may progress to severe liver conditions. Managing diabetes and adopting a healthy lifestyle can help prevent and manage NAFLD.

Can type 2 diabetes be a sign of weak bones?

Not exactly. Type 2 diabetes is linked to a higher risk of bone health problems, but it doesn't directly indicate weak bones. Factors like insulin resistance, inflammation, certain medications, obesity, vitamin D deficiency, hormonal changes, and elevated blood sugar levels can contribute to bone health issues in people with type 2 diabetes. Taking steps to manage these factors can help support bone health.

Can type 2 diabetes cause heart problems?

It can. Type 2 diabetes can increase the risk of heart problems by promoting artery plaque buildup (atherosclerosis). This can result in high blood pressure, disrupting lipid levels, triggering inflammation, damaging small blood vessels, affecting nerve control of the heart, increasing blood clotting, and contributing to heart failure. Managing diabetes through lifestyle changes and medical care can help mitigate these risks.

Does high cholesterol cause type 2 diabetes?

Not exactly. High cholesterol doesn't directly cause type 2 diabetes, but it can increase the risk due to its connection with insulin resistance and related factors like obesity and metabolic syndrome.

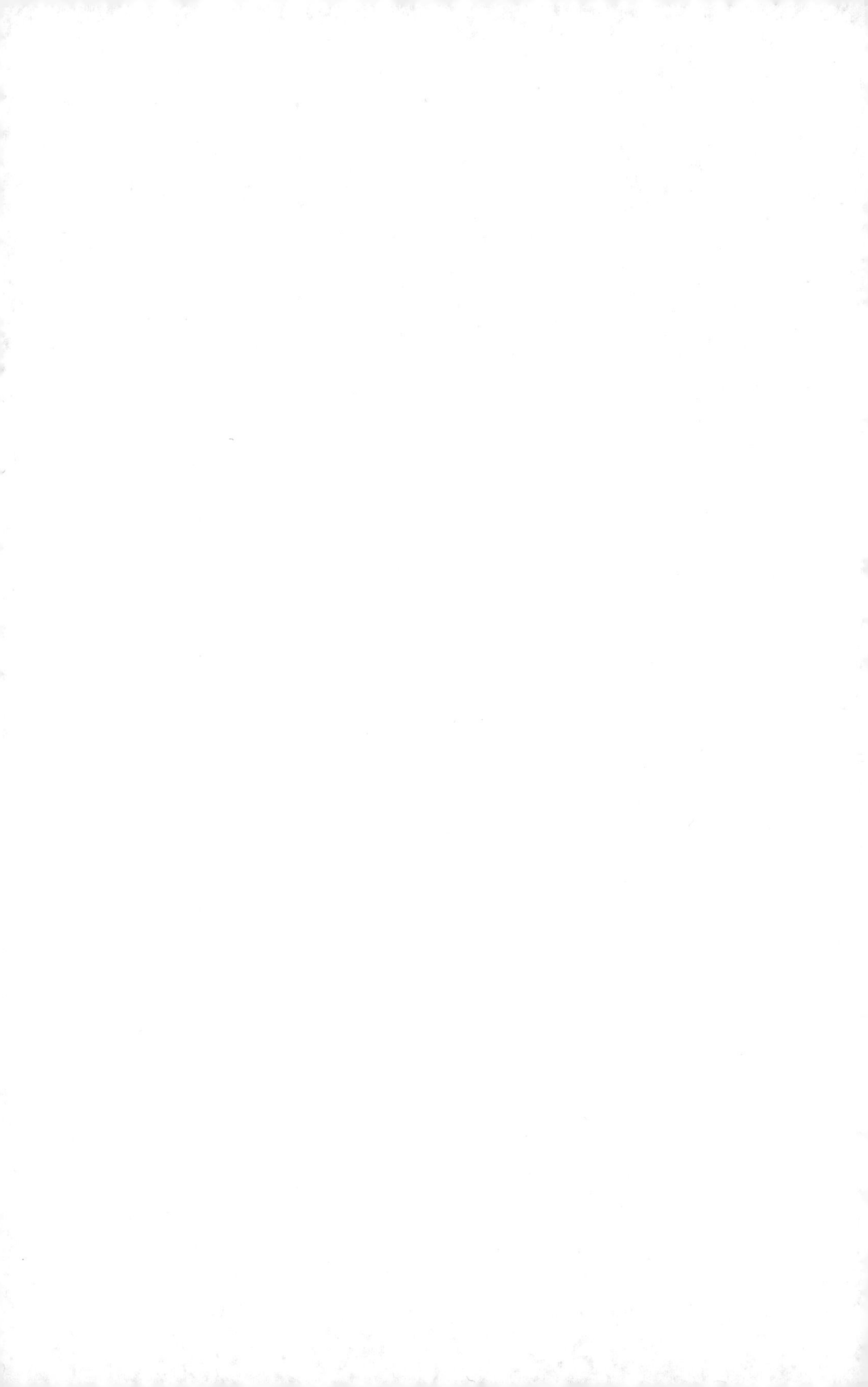

www.ingramcontent.com/pod-product-compliance
Lightning Source LLC
Chambersburg PA
CBHW070755260726
48660CB00007B/3137